Certain necessary directions, as well for the cure of the plague, as for preventing the infection: with many easy medicines ... Set down by the College of Physicians. ...

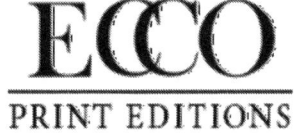

Certain necessary directions, as well for the cure of the plague, as for preventing the infection: with many easy medicines ... Set down by the College of Physicians. ...
Multiple Contributors, See Notes
ESTCID: T097324
Reproduction from British Library
Originally published in 1638 as: Certain necessary directions, aswell for the cure of the plague, as for preventing the infection.
Edinburgh : London, printed 1665: and re-printed at Edinburgh, 1721.
36p. ; 8°

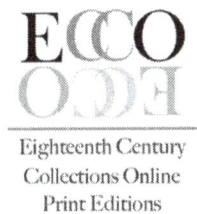

Eighteenth Century
Collections Online
Print Editions

Gale ECCO Print Editions

Relive history with *Eighteenth Century Collections Online*, now available in print for the independent historian and collector. This series includes the most significant English-language and foreign-language works printed in Great Britain during the eighteenth century, and is organized in seven different subject areas including literature and language; medicine, science, and technology; and religion and philosophy. The collection also includes thousands of important works from the Americas.

The eighteenth century has been called "The Age of Enlightenment." It was a period of rapid advance in print culture and publishing, in world exploration, and in the rapid growth of science and technology – all of which had a profound impact on the political and cultural landscape. At the end of the century the American Revolution, French Revolution and Industrial Revolution, perhaps three of the most significant events in modern history, set in motion developments that eventually dominated world political, economic, and social life.

In a groundbreaking effort, Gale initiated a revolution of its own: digitization of epic proportions to preserve these invaluable works in the largest online archive of its kind. Contributions from major world libraries constitute over 175,000 original printed works. Scanned images of the actual pages, rather than transcriptions, recreate the works *as they first appeared.*

Now for the first time, these high-quality digital scans of original works are available via print-on-demand, making them readily accessible to libraries, students, independent scholars, and readers of all ages.

For our initial release we have created seven robust collections to form one the world's most comprehensive catalogs of 18th century works.

Initial Gale ECCO Print Editions collections include:

> ### *History and Geography*
> Rich in titles on English life and social history, this collection spans the world as it was known to eighteenth-century historians and explorers. Titles include a wealth of travel accounts and diaries, histories of nations from throughout the world, and maps and charts of a world that was still being discovered. Students of the War of American Independence will find fascinating accounts from the British side of conflict.

Social Science
Delve into what it was like to live during the eighteenth century by reading the first-hand accounts of everyday people, including city dwellers and farmers, businessmen and bankers, artisans and merchants, artists and their patrons, politicians and their constituents. Original texts make the American, French, and Industrial revolutions vividly contemporary.

Medicine, Science and Technology
Medical theory and practice of the 1700s developed rapidly, as is evidenced by the extensive collection, which includes descriptions of diseases, their conditions, and treatments. Books on science and technology, agriculture, military technology, natural philosophy, even cookbooks, are all contained here.

Literature and Language
Western literary study flows out of eighteenth-century works by Alexander Pope, Daniel Defoe, Henry Fielding, Frances Burney, Denis Diderot, Johann Gottfried Herder, Johann Wolfgang von Goethe, and others. Experience the birth of the modern novel, or compare the development of language using dictionaries and grammar discourses.

Religion and Philosophy
The Age of Enlightenment profoundly enriched religious and philosophical understanding and continues to influence present-day thinking. Works collected here include masterpieces by David Hume, Immanuel Kant, and Jean-Jacques Rousseau, as well as religious sermons and moral debates on the issues of the day, such as the slave trade. The Age of Reason saw conflict between Protestantism and Catholicism transformed into one between faith and logic -- a debate that continues in the twenty-first century.

Law and Reference
This collection reveals the history of English common law and Empire law in a vastly changing world of British expansion. Dominating the legal field is the *Commentaries of the Law of England* by Sir William Blackstone, which first appeared in 1765. Reference works such as almanacs and catalogues continue to educate us by revealing the day-to-day workings of society.

Fine Arts
The eighteenth-century fascination with Greek and Roman antiquity followed the systematic excavation of the ruins at Pompeii and Herculaneum in southern Italy; and after 1750 a neoclassical style dominated all artistic fields. The titles here trace developments in mostly English-language works on painting, sculpture, architecture, music, theater, and other disciplines. Instructional works on musical instruments, catalogs of art objects, comic operas, and more are also included.

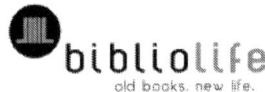

The BiblioLife Network

This project was made possible in part by the BiblioLife Network (BLN), a project aimed at addressing some of the huge challenges facing book preservationists around the world. The BLN includes libraries, library networks, archives, subject matter experts, online communities and library service providers. We believe every book ever published should be available as a high-quality print reproduction; printed on-demand anywhere in the world. This insures the ongoing accessibility of the content and helps generate sustainable revenue for the libraries and organizations that work to preserve these important materials.

The following book is in the "public domain" and represents an authentic reproduction of the text as printed by the original publisher. While we have attempted to accurately maintain the integrity of the original work, there are sometimes problems with the original work or the micro-film from which the books were digitized. This can result in minor errors in reproduction. Possible imperfections include missing and blurred pages, poor pictures, markings and other reproduction issues beyond our control. Because this work is culturally important, we have made it available as part of our commitment to protecting, preserving, and promoting the world's literature.

GUIDE TO FOLD-OUTS MAPS and OVERSIZED IMAGES

The book you are reading was digitized from microfilm captured over the past thirty to forty years. Years after the creation of the original microfilm, the book was converted to digital files and made available in an online database.

In an online database, page images do not need to conform to the size restrictions found in a printed book. When converting these images back into a printed bound book, the page sizes are standardized in ways that maintain the detail of the original. For large images, such as fold-out maps, the original page image is split into two or more pages

Guidelines used to determine how to split the page image follows:

• Some images are split vertically; large images require vertical and horizontal splits.
• For horizontal splits, the content is split left to right.
• For vertical splits, the content is split from top to bottom.
• For both vertical and horizontal splits, the image is processed from top left to bottom right.

Certain necessary
DIRECTIONS,
As well for the
CURE
OF THE
PLAGUE,
As for preventing the
Infection:
WITH
Many easy MEDICINES of small Charge, very profitable to His Majesty's Subjects.

Set down by the College of Physicians.

By the King's Majesty's special Command.

LONDON, Printed 1665: And Reprinted at Edinburgh, 1721.

AN ADVICE

Set down by

The College of Physicians.

By His Majesty's special Command.

Containing certain necessary Directions, as well for the Cure of the PLAGUE, as for preventing the Infection; with many easy Medicines, and of small Charge, the Use whereof may be very profitable to His Majesty's Subjects.

I. *Doctors, Apothecaries, and Chirurgeons.*

THE Church-Orders for Prayers being first observed as in former Times, it might be desired, that by the Government of the City there be appointed six or four Doctors at least, who may apply them-

themselves to the Cure of the Infected, and that these Doctors be Stipendiaries to the City for their Lives; and that to each Doctor there be assigned two Apothecaries and three Chirurgeons, who are also to be stipended by the City; that so due and true Care may be taken in all Things, that the People perish not without Help, and that the Infection spread not, while none take particular Care to resist it, as in *Paris*, *Venice*, and *Padua*, and many other Cities

And if any Doctor, Apothecary, or Chirurgeon stipended by the City shall happen to die in the Service of the Attendance of the Plague, then their Widows surviving shall have their Pensions during their Lives

II. *Prevention of propagating the Infection from Place to Place.*

AS the Provision already made by Authority, upon Occasion, of prohibiting Persons and Goods coming from foreign Countries and Places infected, to be landed, for fourty Days, is most rational, for preventing the bringing in of the Contagion from any such Places; so it is advisable, that some suitable Provision be made in relation *the Physicians*

lation to Persons within the kingdom, who may remove or travel from Places much infected, to sound, as, That none might travel without Certificate of Health; that Persons justly suspected might not be suffered to enter such Places free from Infection, but speedily sent away, or kept in some House or Houses set apart to receive such Persons (with Accommodation of Necessaries) for forty or thirty Days at least, till their Soundness might appear; And that any Goods coming from the like Places might be opened and aired, before received into Houses free and clear.

III. *Prevention of dispersing the Contagion amongst Persons.*

IT is adviseable, That all needless Concourses of People be prohibited; That the Poor be relieved and set at work, and Beggers not suffered to go about; That all Sale of corrupt Provision for Food be restrained, That Streets and Houses be diligently and carefully as may be, kept clean, the Streets washed and cooled as much as may be, by the plentiful running of the Conduits and Water otherwise procured. And it were to be wished, that
Vaul

The Advice of

Vaults for Privies might be emptied only in Winter: And that Soap-suds and Liquors wherein foul Clothes are washed or rinsed, might, as much as may be, be otherwise conveyed, than through the Streets and Gutters, or washed away with Plenty of Water.

It were also to be wished, That the Slaughter-houses were utterly put from out the Liberties of the City, being in themselves very offensive; And that Funnels in Church-vaults be considered of, and the Depth of Graves, and the putting of Quick-Lime into them, and the infected buried without the City.

IV. *To be cautelous upon any Suspicion.*

IT is to be presumed, because every one desireth his own Liberty, that none will give notice of any Suspicion of the Plague against themselves; wherefore that must be the Overseers Care, upon any Notice or Suspicion of Infection, by the Help of the Doctors, Chirurgeons, Keepers or Searchers, to find out the Truth thereof, and so to proceed accordingly, but not to depend upon the Testimony of Women-searchers alone.

V. *Di-*

V. Directions for the Searchers.

1. They are to take Notice whether there be any Swellings, Risings, or Botch under the Ear, about the Neck, on either Side, or under the Arm-pits of either Side, or the Groins, and of its hardness, and whether broken or unbroken.

2. Whether there be any Blains which may arise in any part of the Body in the form of a Blister, much bigger than the Small Pox, of a straw-colour, or livid colour, which latter is the worser; either of them hath a reddish Circuit, something swollen round about it, which Circuit remains after the Blister is broken, encompassing the Sore.

3. Whether there be any Carbuncle, which is something like the Blain, but more fiery and corrosive, easily eating deep into the Flesh, and sometimes having a black Crust upon it, but always compassed about with a very fiery red (or livid) flat and hard Tumour, about a finger-breadth more or less: This and the Blain may appear in any part of the Body.

4 Whether there be any Tokens, which are Spots arising upon the Skin, chiefly about

bout the Breast and Back, but sometimes also in other Parts, their Colour is something various, sometimes more reddish, sometimes inclining a little toward a faint blue, and sometimes brownish mixt with blue; the red ones have often a purple-circle about them, the brownish, a reddish.

5. Whether the Neck and other Limbs are rigid or stiff, or more flexible and limber than in other dead Bodies

VI. *The Care to be taken when a House is visited.*

THat upon the Discovery of the Infection in any House, there be presently Means used to preserve the Whole, as well as to cure the Infected: And that no sick Person be removed out of any House, tho' to another of his own, without notice thereof to be given to the Overseers, and to be by them approved; or if the whole be to be removed, that notice be given to the Overseers of their Remove, and that Caution be given that they shall not wander about till they be found.

The House that is known to be infected, tho' none be dead therein, to be shut up, and carefully kept watched by more trusty Men.

the Physicians. 9

Men than ordinary Warders, till a time after the Party be well recovered, and that time to be forty Days at the least, or rather remove them all immediately to the Pest-houses.

VII. *Caution about Apparel and Housholdstuff.*

THat no Apparel or Housholdstuff be removed, or sold out of the infected House, for six Months after the Infection is ceased in the House; And that all the Brokers, and inferior Cryers for Apparel be restrained in that behalf, and such Apparel or Housholdstuff to be aired and fumed.

VIII. *Correction of the Air.*

FIres made in the Streets often, and good Fires kept in and about the Houses of such as are visited, and their Neighbours, may correct the infectious Air; as also frequent discharging of Guns.

Also Fumes of these following Materials; Rosin, Pitch, Tar, Turpentine, Frank-Incense, Myrrhe, Amber, The Woods of Juniper, Cypress, Cedar; The Leaves of

B Bays,

Bays, Rosemary; to which, especially to the less grateful sented, may be added somewhat of *Labdanum, Storax, Benzoin, Lignum aloes*, one or more of these, as they are at hand, or may be procured, are to be put upon Coals, and consumed with the least Flame that may be, in Rooms, Houses, Churches, or other Places.

Brimstone burnt plentifully in any Room or Place, tho' ill to be endured for the present, may effectually correct the Air for the future.

Vapours from Vineger exhaled in any Room may have the like Efficacy, especially after it hath been impregnated, by infusing or steeping in it any one or more of these Ingredients, Wormwood, Angelica, Master-wort, Bay-leaves, Rosemary, Rue, Sage, *Scordium*, or Water-germander, Valerium, or Setwall-root, Zedoarie, Camphire. To which Vineger also, to render it less ungrateful, may be added Rosewater, to a fourth or third part: These are cooler, and so more proper for hot Seasons.

The Vapour of Vineger raised by slaking of Lime in it, may effectually correct the Air near about it.

Take Salt-peter, Amber, Brimstone, of each two parts, of Juniper one part; mix them

them in a Powder, put thereof upon a red hot Iron, or Coals, a little at once.

IX. *Perfuming of Apparel.*

THis also may preserve from Infection, being done by some of the more grateful of the dry Fumes of the Gumms, &c. before mentioned to be burnt; and between whiles frequent shifting and airing of Apparel may be, especially by the Fire, or in the Sun, the more effectual, this to be done the rather, if one hath come in Danger of Infection.

X. *By carrying about of Perfumes.*

SUch as are to go abroad, shall do well to carry Rue, Angelica, Masterwort, Myrrh, Scordium, or Water germander, Wormwood, Valerian, or Setwall-root, Virginian-snake-root, or Zedoarie in their Hands to smell to, and of those they may hold or chew a little in their Mouths as they go in the Streets; They may anoint their Nostrils with Oyl of Amber, or Balsam of Sulphur; especially if they be afraid of any Place: Fear, as well as Presumption, being hurtful.

The Advice of

Take Rue one handful, stamp it in a Mortar, put thereto Vineger enough to moisten it, mix them well, then strain out the Juice, wet a piece of Spunge, or a Toast of brown Bread therein, tie it in a thin Cloth, bear it about to smell to.

Take the Root of Angelica beaten grosly, the weight of six pence, of Rue, and Wormwood, of each the weight of four pence, Setwall the weight of three pence; bruise these, then steep them in a little Wine Vineger, tie them in a linnen Cloth, which they may carry in their Hands, or put it into a Juniper-box full of Holes to smell to.

XI. Or they may use this Pomander.

Take Angelica, Rue, Zedoarie, of each half a Dram, Myrrh two Drams, Camphire six Grains, Wax and *Labdanum* of each two Drams, more or less, as shall be thought fit to mix with the other things; make hereof a Ball to carry about you; you may easily make a Hole in it, and so wear it about your Neck with a String.

XII. The

XII. *The richer Sort may make Use of this Pomander.*

TAke Citron-pills, Angelica-seeds, Zedoary, Red-rose-leaves, of each half a Dram, yellow Saunders, *Lignum aloes*, of each one Scruple, *Galla Moschata* four Scruples, Storax, Benzoin, of each one Dram, Camphire six Grains, *Laudanum* three Drams, Gum-Tragacanth dissolved in Rosewater, enough to make it up into a Pomander, put thereto six Drops of Spirit of Roses, inclose it in an Ivory-box, or wear it about your Neck.

XIII. *By inward Medicines.*

LEt none go fasting forth, every one according as they can procure, let them take some such thing as may resist Putrefaction.

Some may take Garlick with Butter, a Clove, two or three, according as it shall agree with their Bodies; some may take fasting, some of the Electuary with *Figs* and *Rue* hereafter expressed, some may use *London* Treacle, the weight of eight pence in the Morning, taking more or less, according

ding to the Age of the Party; after one Hour let them eat some other Breakfast, as Bread and Butter with some Leaves of Rue or Sage moistned with Vineger, and in the heat of Summer of Sorrel or Wood-sorrel.

Pure Water with so much Salt as may be but tasted, or well born; or with Flour of Brimstone, or common Brimstone boyl'd in it, an Ounce in three Pints, to a Quart, a Draught being taken every Morning, hath proved effectual and successful.

To steep Rue, Wormwood, or Sage all Night in their Drink, and to drink a good Draught in the Morning fasting, is very wholesome, or to drink a Draught of such Drink after the taking of any of the Preservatives will be very good.

Take of Sage bruised well two handfuls, of Wormwood one handful, of Rue half a handful, put them into a Jugg of four Quarts, put to them of mild Beer ready to drink four Quarts; in the Morning let every one of the Family drink a Draught of it fasting, together eating after it Bread and Butter.

Take of the Roots of *Petasitis*, or Butter-burre, six Ounces, Roots of Elecampane, Masterwort, and Angelica, of each 1. Ounce and half, Leaves of Meadow-sweet, *Scordium*,

Scordium, Bawm, of each two handfuls, Rue and Wormwood of each one handful, Citron (or Limon) peel, Nutmeg, of each half an Ounce, of Juniper-berries ripe and pulpey two Ounces, of Carduus-seed one Ounce; All duly prepared by cutting and bruising, are to be mixed and put into a Bag, to infuse in six Gallons of Ale or Beer, whereof may be drunk a Draught every Morning and Evening; and at Meals it may be mingled with ordinary Beer.

Take of the Conserve of Wood-sorrel two Ounces, of Diascordium two Drams, of the Flour of Brimstone very finely ground one Dram, of Saffron three Grains, of Syrup of Wood-sorrel, as much as is sufficient to make an Electuary. For Prevention, take a Dram every Morning fasting, during the imminent Danger: Let the Party drink after it a Draught of white-wine Posset, with a Spoonful and half of the Plague-water in it in Bed, or of this Water following.

Take of Angelica, *Carduus benedictus*, Sage, *Scordium*, *Petasitis*, or Butter-burre, Bawm, and Plantain, of each four handfuls, of Setwall and Borage of each two handfuls, of Mint one handful, of white-wine two Quarts; distill them in a cold Still, and preserve the Water for Use.

XIV. The

XIV. *The Plague-water of Matthias, or,* Aqua Epidemica.

TAke the Roots of Tormentil, Angelica, Peony, Zedoarie, Liquorish, Elecampane, of each half an Ounce, the Leaves of Sage, *Scordium,* Celandine, Rue, Rosemary, Wormwood, *Ros solis,* Mugwort, Burnet, Dragons, Scabious, Agrimony, Bawm, *Carduus,* Betony, Centery the less, Marygolds Leaves and Flowers, of each one handful; Let them all be cut, bruised, and infused three Days in eight Pints of Whitewine in the Month of *May,* and distilled.

Take of *London*-Treacle two Ounces, of Conserve of Wood-sorrel three Ounces, of the temperate Cordial species half an Ounce, of Syrup of Limons enough to make all an Electuary. Of this may be taken a Dram and half for Prevention, and the double Quantity for Cure.

Steep Juniper-berries in Vineger for a Night, let the Vineger be exhaled off; eat thereof at Pleasure.

An Electuary of Bole-Armeniack, as much as you please; or of the Powders whereof the Treacle *Diatesseron* is made, mixed up with Syrup of Vineger; or an Electuary of Zedoarie, *the Physicians.*

Zedoarie, with Syrup of Limons, are easily made, and very effectual, being taken as the former.

In all Summer-plagues it shall be good to use Sorrel-sawce to be eaten in the Morning with Bread, and in the Fall of the Leaf to use the Juice of Barbaries with Bread also.

XV. Mithridates *his Medicine of Figs.*

Take of good Figs, and Walnut-kernels, of each twenty four, Rue picked two handfuls, of Salt half an Ounce or somewhat better. First, stamp your Figs and Walnuts well together in a Stone-mortar, then add your Rue, and last of all your Salt, mix them exceeding well ; take of this Mixture every Morning fasting, the Weight of sixteen pence, to Children and weak Bodies less.

XVI. *Or this will be effectual also.*

Take twenty Walnuts, pill them, Figs fifteen, Rue a good handful, Tormentil-roots three Drams, Bole-Armoniack a Dram and a half. First stamp your Roots, then your Figs and Seeds, then add your
Walnuts,

Walnuts, then put to your Rue and Bole and with them put thereto six Drams o *London*-Treacle, and two or three Spoonful of Wine-vineger, mix them well in a Stone mortar, and take of this every Morning the Quantity of a good Nutmeg fasting. They that have Cause to go much abroad may take as much more in the Evening two Hours before Supper.

Take of Figs half a Pound, of Walnut-kernels two Ounces, of dried Rue leaves one Ounce, of Salt half an Ounce, of the Root of *Petasitis* six Drams, *Contrayerva* root, Virginian Snake-root, Salt of *Prunella*, of each a Dram and half, of Zedoarie a Dram, of Sugar dissolved in Vineger to a Syrup, enough to make all into an Electuary.

Hereof may be taken a Dram or the Quantity of a Nutmeg every Morning and Evening.

XVII. *For Women with Child, Children, and such as cannot take bitter things, use this.*

TAke Conserve of Red-roses, Conserve of Wood-sorrel, of each two Ounces, Conserves of Borage, of Sage-flowers, of each six Drams, Bole-Armoniack, Shavings of of Harts-horn, Sorrel-seeds, of each two Drams, yellow or white Saunders half a Dram, Saffron one Scruple, Syrup of Wood-sorrel, enough to make it a moist Electuary; mix them well, take so much as a Chesnut at a Time, once or twice a Day, as you shall find Cause.

XVIII. *For the richer Sort.*

Take the Shavings of Harts-horn, of Pearl, of Coral, Tormentil-roots, Zedoarie, true *Terra Sigillata,* of each one Dram, Citron pills, yellow, white and red Saunders, of each half a Dram, white Amber, Hyacinth-stone prepared, of each two Scruples, Bezoar-stone of the East, Unicorns horn, of each four and twenty Grains, Citron and Orange-peels candied, of each three Drams, *Lignum Aloes* one Scruple, white Sugar-candie twice the Weight of all the rest; mix them well, being made into a Dredge-powder. Take the Weight of twelve pence at a Time every Morning fasting, and also in the Evening about five a Clock, or an Hour before Supper.

With these Powders and Sugar there may be made Lozenges, or *Manus Christi's,* and with convenient Conserves they may be made into Electuaries. All which, and many more for their Health, they may have by the Advice and Directions of their own Physicians; or, as we hope, Physicians will not be wanting to direct them as they may have need, to the Poor for Charity sake.

They may also use Bezoar-water, or Treacle-water distilled, compounded by the Physicians of *London*, and known by the Name of *Aqua Theriacalis stillatitia*, which they may use simply; or they may mix them also with all their Antidotes, as Occasion shall require.

Take of Amber-gryse a Scruple, dissolve it in four Ounces of the best Spirit of Sack; take hereof every Morning a Scruple, with Crumbs of White-bread and Sugar of Roses. Balsam of Sulphur to four or five Drops, or *Elixir Proprietatis* to twenty or thirty Drops, in Wine, or Water and Sugar, may be effectual.

The use of *London*-Treacle is good, both to preserve from the Sickness, as also to cure the Sick, being taken upon the first Apprehension in a greater Quantity, as to a Man two Drams, but less to a weak Body, or a Child, in Cardnus or Dragon-water.

Take of the finest clear Aloes you can buy, of Cinnamon, of Myrrh, of each of these

these the weight of three *French* Crowns, or of Two and twenty pence of our Money, of Cloves, Mace, *Lignum Aloes*, of Mastick, of Bole-Oriental, of each of these half an Ounce; mingle them together, and beat them into a very fine Powder, of the which take every Morning fasting the weight of a Groat in White-wine deluyed with Water.

Take a dry Fig, and open it, and put the Kernel of a Walnut into the same, being cut very small, three or four Leaves of Rue, commonly called Herb-Grace, a Corn of Salt; then rost the Fig and eat it warm, fast three or four Hours after it, and use this twice in the Week.

Take the Powder of Tormentil the weight of six pence, with Sorrel or Scabious-water in Summer, and in the Winter with the Water of Valerian, or common Drink, wherein hath been infused the forenamed Herbs.

Or else, in one Day they may take a little Worm-wood and Valerian, with a Grain of Salt; in another Day they may take seven or eight Berries of Juniper dried, and put in Powder, and taking the same with common Drink, or with Drink in which Wormwood and Rue hath been steeped all Night.

Also the Treacle called *Diatesseron*, which is made but of four things of light Price, easy

ſy to be had: The Ingredients are, Gentian, Bay-berries, Myrrh, and *Ariſtolochia* the round, in equal proportion, made into an Electuary with three Times the weight of Honey.

Alſo the Root of *Elecampane* taken in Powder with Drink.

Likewiſe a Piece of Orris-root kept in the Mouth as Men paſs in the Streets.

Take ſix Leaves of Sorrel, waſh them with Water and Vineger, let them lie in the ſaid Water and Vineger a while, then eat them faſting, and keep in your Mouth and chew now and then either Setwall, or the Root of Angelica, or a little Cinnamon, or four Grains of Myrrh, or ſo much of Rattle-ſnake root: Goats Rue may be eaten in Salads, or the Juice or Decoction thereof in Broth or Poſſet-drink, may be ſo uſed to very good purpoſe.

XIX. *Iſſues.*

SUch as are tied to neceſſary Attendance on the Infected, as alſo ſuch as live in Viſited Houſes, ſhall do well to cauſe Iſſues to be made in their Arms or Legs, or both, as the Phyſician ſhall think fit.

XX. *Bleed-*

XX. *Bleeding, Purging, Vomiting.*

These three great Remedies rarely have place in the Plague, but are generally dangerous, (and most of all, purging by any strong Medicines) and therefore not to be used but upon some extraordinary, urgent, indicant or just Occasion, and with the greatest Caution, which only an able Physician can judge of, and therefore, no Advice in general can be given: Only if any Person be taken sick upon a full stomach, from eating lately before, or Meat undigested; It is advisable that such Person discharge or get the Stomach emptied with all Speed by a large Quantity of Carduus, or plain Posset-drink, or warm Water, provoking by a Feather or Finger in the Throat as is usual. And when need requires, to open or keep soluble the Body, the Pills of *Rufus,* commonly called *Pestilential-Pills,* are the best and most proper to be used.

XXI. *Me-*

XXI. *Medicines expulsive.*

THE Poison is expelled best by Sweating, provoked by Posset-ale, made with Fennel and Marygolds in Winter, and with Sorrel, Buglofs and Borage in Summer; with the which in both Times they must mingle *London* Treacle the Weight of two Drams, and so lay themselves with all Quietness to sweat.

For those that are able to bear it, this Course is effectual, and hath proved successful. Let the Party take a large Dose of any of these Cordials that is next at Hand, that is to say, of *London*-Treacle, or Diascordium, of either half an Ounce, or of Mithridate a quarter of an Ounce, or of *Venice*-Treacle half a quarter, or a quarter of an Ounce at most, in a Draught of Posset-drink made with White-wine, or Vineger, then let him be put to bed to sweat, well covered, in a Blanket, without his Shirt, for 24 Hours, every sixth Hour renewing his Cordial, but in half the Quantity formerly directed, between whiles refreshing him with Posset-drink, Oatmeal-caudle, or thin Broths made Ge's wife, or Harts-horn Gelly.

If the Person be unapt to sweat, lay two

or three Bricks, quenched in Vineger, wrapped up in a woollen Cloth, to his Body to promote it.

At the same Time that he applieth himself to sweat, he must apply Blisters to the Parts of his Body, as is elsewhere directed; Or Rowelling with Bryony, Hellebor, or Setterwort roots, doth exceeding well on the same Occasion.

Take of Angelica root two Ounces, of Tormentil-root an Ounce and half, make a Decoction in two Pints of Water to a Pint and half, add three Ounces of Juice of Lemon, or an Ounce and half of Vineger; let the sick drink a Draught as he can bear, and repete it at two or three Hours Distance.

Take of Mithridate to the Quantity of two Drams, or of *London* Treacle, or of Diascordium to three Drams, or of *Venice*-Treacle to a Dram and half, dissolve either of them in a quarter of a Pint of Vineger, and drink it.

Take of *Venice*-Treacle a Dram, Diascordium two Scruples, Salt of Wormwood, Crabs eyes, of each a Scruple, Treacle-water an Ounce and half, Juice of Lemons, or Vineger two Ounces, for one Dose.

For the Cure of the Infected upon the first Apprehension; Burr-seeds, Cochineal, Powder

der of Harts-horn, Citron-seeds, one or more of them, with a few Grains of Camphire, are good to be given in Carduus or Dragon-water, or with some Treacle water.

Take of White-wine Vinegar from half a quarter to a quarter of a Pint, mixed with Salt, from twenty Grains to forty, drink it warm, and sweat upon it. Or take the Juice of fresh Cow-dung, strained with Vineger, from three Spoonfuls to seven.

XXII. *Avicen's Medicine.*

Take of Bole-Armeniack a Dram, of Juice of Orange half an Ounce, of White-wine an Ounce, of Red-Rose-Water two Ounces, mix them, and give it assoon as the Party suspects the Disease, if it be vomited, repete it again; if vomited again, repete it the second Time.

Take of Burr-seeds half a Dram, of Cochineal half a Scruple, of Camphire six Grains; mix these with two Ounces of Carduus, or Dragon-water, half an Ounce of Treacle water, Syrup of Wood sorrel, a Spoonful, mix these, give it the Patient warm, cover him to sweat; you may give him a second Draught after twelve Hours, Let him drink no cold drink, This Posset-drink,

drink, or the like, will be good to give the Vinegar liberally.

Take Citron-seeds six or eight shavings, of Harts-horn half a dram, London-Treacle one Dram, mix them with two Ounces of Carduus-water, or with three Ounces of the prescribed Posset-drink, drink it warm, and so lie to sweat.

Take Sorrel Water, five or six Spoonfuls, Treacle Water one Spoonful, London-Treacle one Dram and a half, mix them well, give it warm, and so let the Patient to sweat.

Take Tormentil, and Celandine-roots, of each four Ounces, Scabious and Rue, of each one handful and an half, White-wine Vinegar three Pints, boyl these till one Pint be wasted, strain out the Liquor, which reserve for the Use of the Infected: let it be taken thus.

Take of this Liquor, and of Carduus-water, of each one Ounce and an half, London-Treacle one Dram and an half, Bole-Armenick half a Scruple, put thereto a little Sugar, mix them well, let the Party drink it warm, and cover him to sweat.

XXIII. *In Summer this is good.*

Take the *Juice* of Wood-sorrel two Ounces, Juice of Lemons one Ounce,

Ounce, Diascordium one Dram, Cinnamon six Grains, Vineger half an Ounce; give it warm, and lay the sick Party to sweat; use this in Case of Fluxes of the Belly, or want of rest.

Take of Treacle of *Andromachus* or *Venice*-Treacle, from half a Dram to a Dram; or of *Electuar. um de Ovo*, from a Scruple to half a Dram, in warm Posset Ale, assoon as you suspect your self infected, going to Bed, and sweating upon it.

Take of the Roots of Butterburre, the inner Bark of Ash, of each a Pound; Rue, Scordium, Angelica, Meadow-Sweet, Dragons, Carduus, of each three handfuls, White-wine and Vineger of each two Quarts; let them infuse for a Day or two, and after be distilled; adding to the rest (if to be had) six handfuls of the green Rhinds of Walnuts: Let the Water be sweetned with Syrup of Wood-Sorrel, adding to two Quarts half a Dram of Camphire, and three Drams of Spirit of Sulphur. This Water may be given from two Ounces to four.

Take of the Roots of Butterburre eight Ounces, let them be infused in a Gallon of Ale for four and twenty Hours, and then distilled in a Limbeck, add to the distilled Water six Pints of a strong Decoction of

Carduus,

the Physicians.

Carduus, and in these Liquors infuse Roots of Butterburre, Masterwort, Angelica, Valerian, of each six Ounces, Elecampane-root an Ounce, Leaves of *Scordium*, Bawm, of each three handfuls; of Juniper-berries half an Ounce, After four and twenty Hours infusing in a Bath or hot Water, make a second Distillation. Of this Water may be given three or four Ounces with warm Posset-Ale.

Take of the Root Butterburre, otherwise called Pestilent-wort, one Ounce, of the Root of Great-Valerian a Quarter of an Ounce, of Sorrel an handful, boil all these in a Quart of Water to a Pint, then strain it, and put thereto two Spoonfuls of Vineger, and dissolve in it two Ounces of good Sugar: Let the Infected drink of this, so hot as he may suffer it, a good Draught, and if he chance to cast it up again, let him take the same Quantity straightway upon it, and provoke himself to sweat.

Take of the Powder of good Bay-berries, the Husk taken away from them before they be dried, or of Ivy-berries well dried, a Spoonful; let the Patient drink this well mingled in a Draught of good stale Ale or Beer, or with a Draught of White-wine, and go to Bed, and cast himself into a Sweat, and forbear Sleep.

Take

Take the inward Bark of the Ash-tree one Pound, of Walnuts with the green outward Shells to the Number of fifty, cut these small, of Scabious, of Vervin, of each a handful, of Saffron two Drams, pour upon these the strongest Vinegar you can get, four Pints, let them a little boil together upon a very soft Fire, and then stand in a very close Pot well stopt all a Night upon the Embers, after distil them with a soft Fire, and receive the Water close kept. Give unto the Patient laid in Bed and well covered with Clothes, two Ounces of this Water to drink, and let him be provoked to sweat; and every eight Hours, during the space of four and twenty Hours, give him the same Quantity to drink.

Care must be taken in the Use of these Sweating Cordials, that the Party infected sweat two or three Hours, or rather much longer, if he have Strength, and sleep not till the Sweat be over, and that he have been well wiped with warm Linen, and when he hath been dryed, let him wash his Mouth with Water and Vinegar warm, and let his Face and Hands be washed with the same. When these things are done, give him a good Draught of Broth made with Chicken, or Mutton, with Rosemary, Thyme, Sorrel,

Suc-

Succory, and Marygolds; or else Water-grewel, with Rosemary, and Winter-Savory, or Thyme, Panado seasoned with Verjuice, or Juice of Wood-Sorrel: For their Drink, let it be small Beer warmed, with a Tost, or Water boyled with Carraway-seed, Carduus seed, and a Crust of Bread, or such Posset-drink as is mentioned before in the second Medicine; after some Nutriment let them sleep or rest, often washing their Mouth with Water and Vineger.

These Cordials must be repeated once in eight, ten, or twelve Hours at the farthest.

If the Party infested vomit up his Medicine, then repete it presently.

XXIV. *Medicines External.*

VEsicatories applied behind the Ears, about the Wrists, near the Arm-pits, on the Inside of the Thighs, and near the Groins, will draw forth the Venome.

For the swelling under the Ears, Arm-pits, or in the Groins, they must be always drawn forth and ripened, and broke with all speed.

These Tumours, and much more the Carbuncles and Blains do require the Care and Skill of the expert Chirurgeon: but not to

leave

leave the poorer Sort destitute of good Remedies; these following are very good

Pull off the Feathers from the Tails of living Cocks, Hens, Pigeons, or Chickens, and holding their Bills, hold them hard to the Botch or Swelling, and so keep them to that Part until they die, and by this Means draw out the Poison: It is good to apply a Cupping-Glass, or Embers in a Dish, with a handful of Sorrel upon the Embers.

XXV. *To break the Tumor.*

TAke a great Onion, hollow it, put into it a Fig, Rue cut small, and a Dram of *Venice* Treacle, put it close stopt in a wet Paper, and rost it in the Embers, apply it hot unto the Tumor, lay three or four, one after another, let one lie three Hours.

Or it may be better to rost the Onion and Fig apart, the Onion being kept whole, and then, that all be beaten and mixed together. Take Roots of white Lillies, Figs, Leeks rosted, of each an Ounce, of Line seed half an Ounce, let them be beat together in a Morter, and mixed with six Drams of old sour Leaven, adding as much Oil of Lillies, as may give a due Consistence; Let it be applied to the Tumor till it ripen and break;

which

which last, if it do not in a long Time it may be opened by Incision, or a Caustick applied upon, or a little below it.

Scabious and Sorrel rosted in the Embers, mixt with a little strong Leaven, and some Barrow's-grease, and a little Salt, will draw it and break it.

Take two or three rosted Onions, a Lillieroot or two, rosted, a handful of Scabious rosted, four or five Figs, a Piece of Leaven, and a little Rue, stamp all these together; if it be too dry, put to it of Oil of Lillies as much as shall be needful, or so much Salt Butter; make a Pultess, apply it hot, after it hath lyen three or four Hours take it off, and burn it, and apply a fresh Pultess of the same, if it prove hard to break, and a little burnt Copperas to the Pultess.

Or this.

TAke the Flowers of Elders two handfuls, Rocket-seed bruised one Ounce, Pigeons Dung three Drams; stamp these together, put to them a little Oil of Lillies, make thereof a Pultess, apply it, and change it as you did the former.

XXVI. To

XXVI. *To draw.*

WHen it is broken to draw it, and heal it, take the Yolk of an Egg, one Ounce of Honey of Roses, Turpentine half an Ounce, Wheat-flour a little, *London*-Treacle a Dram and a half; mix these well, spread it upon Leather, change it twice a Day, or take *Diachylon cum Gummis*.

XXVII. *For the Carbuncle.*

APply an actual or potential Cautery, laying a Defensative of Bole-Armeniack, or *Terra Sigillata* mixed with Vineger, and the White of an Egg, round about the Tumour, but not upon it.

Take three or four Cloves of Garlick, Rue half a handful, four Figs, strong Leven, and the Soot of a Chimney in which Wood hath been burnt, of each half an Ounce, Mustard-seed two Drams, Salt a Dram and a half; stamp these well together, and apply it hot to the Sore; you may put thereto a little Salt Butter, if it be too dry.

Or this.

TAke Leven half an Ounce, Radish-roots, the bigger the better, an Ounce and an half, Mustard-seed two Drams, Onions and Garlick rosted, of each two Drams and an half, *Venice*-Treacle or *Mithridatum* three Drams; mix these in a Morter, apply it hot thrice a Day to the Sore.

But these Sores cannot be well ordered and cured, without the personal Care of a discreet Chirurgion.

Take

Take of Scabious two handfuls, stamp it in a Stone-morter, then put into it of old Swines Grease salted two Ounces, and the Yolk of an Egg; stamp them well together, and lay part of this warm to the Sore.

Take of the Leaves of Mallows, of Camomil-flowers, of each of them a handful, of Linseed beaten into Powder two Ounces, boil the Mallow-leaves first cut, and the Flowers of Camomil in fair Water, standing about a Finger's breadth, boil all them together, until all the Water be almost spent, then put thereunto the Linseed of Wheat flower half a handful, of Swines Grease, the Skins taken away, three Ounces, of Oyl of Lillies two Ounces, stir them still with a Stick, and let them all boil together on a soft Fire without Smoke, until the Water be utterly spent. Beat them all together in a Morter until they be well incorporated, and in feeling, smooth and not rough; then take part thereof hot in a Dish, set upon a Chaffing-dish of Coals, and lay it thick upon a linnen Cloth, applying it to the Sore.

Take a white Onion cut in Pieces, of fresh Butter three Ounces, of Leaven the weight of twelve pence, of Mallows one handful, of Scabious one handful, of Cloves of Garlick the weight of twenty pence. Boil them on the Fire in sufficient Water, and make a Pultess of it, and lay it warm to the Sore.

Another.

Take two handfuls of Valerian, two Ounces of Dane wort, an handful of Smallage or Lovage; seethe them all in Butter and Water, with a few Crumbs of Bread, and make a Pultess thereof, and lay it warm to the Sore till it break.

Another.

The Advice of

Another.

IF you cannot have these Herbs, it is good to lay a Loaf of Bread to it hot, as it cometh out of the Oven (which afterward shall be burnt or buried in the Earth) or the Leaves of Scabious or Sorrel rosted, or two or three Lilly-roots rosted under Embers, beaten and applied.

It will be good to forbear all crude and moist Fruits, as Cucumbers, Melons, Plumbs, Cherries, Peaches, and raw Herbs and Sallads, as Lettice, Spinage, Radish, and such like; or to be moderate in the use of them, mixt with Oyl and Vineger.

Those that are delighted with Chymical Medicines only, may make use of some of these following, being honestly prepared according to the Descriptions of the Authors, and cautiously administred.

Elixir Pestilentiale.
Elixir Proprietatis.
Sulphur album & fixum.
Tinctura auri & Sulphuris fixi incremabilis.
Mixtura Bezoardica.
Extractum Pestilentiale.
Aurum Diaphoreticum.
Aurum vitæ.
Bezoardicum minerale purpurascens.
Bezoardicum minerale diaphoreticum.
Turpetum minerale diaphoreticum.
Aqua gratiæ Dei.
Spiritus Antipestiferus.
Præcipitatus auri diaphoreticus.

FINIS.

www.ingramcontent.com/pod-product-compliance
Ingram Content Group UK Ltd.
Pitfield, Milton Keynes, MK11 3LW, UK
UKHW010657090425
5394UKWH00022B/752